Hemp Oil & You

By:

Ray Tokes

With debate around the medical and recreational use of marijuana now opening up, across America, there's suddenly more freedom to talk openly about the plant and its many benefits.

Contrary to popular belief, the discussion goes much deeper than whether or not people should be able to legally smoke marijuana in their homes.

There is actually avid interest and enthusiasm for cannabis products that are higher in different levels of cannabinoids.

One such product is hemp oil. While it comes from the same plant as marijuana, it contains no THC.

This means that it has no psychotropic qualities, but it does offer a litany of remarkable health benefits. Over the years, the CBD (cannabidiol) in hemp oil has been linked to improvements in everything from dry skin to immune-deficiencies, cancer, acne, poor cholesterol, strokes, heart disease and more.

When people learn about the health benefits of hemp oil for the first time, there is an instant question as to why it is not more widely available.

It seems crazy that such a wondrous substance is not already being prescribed by doctors and used to treat chronic disorders.

However, there has always been a major obstacle limiting the use of hemp oil; its legal connection to the marijuana plant. To clarify, unlike marijuana, the sale and use of hemp oil is completely legal.

This is precisely because hemp oil doesn't contain THC, so it doesn't have the same impact on the brain as marijuana.

For some users, it reportedly provides a calm and relaxed sensation, but there is no fuzziness. The euphoria is felt differently.

It can be used, recreationally, to boost general health and nutrition, treat skin and hair problems, control diabetes symptoms and more.

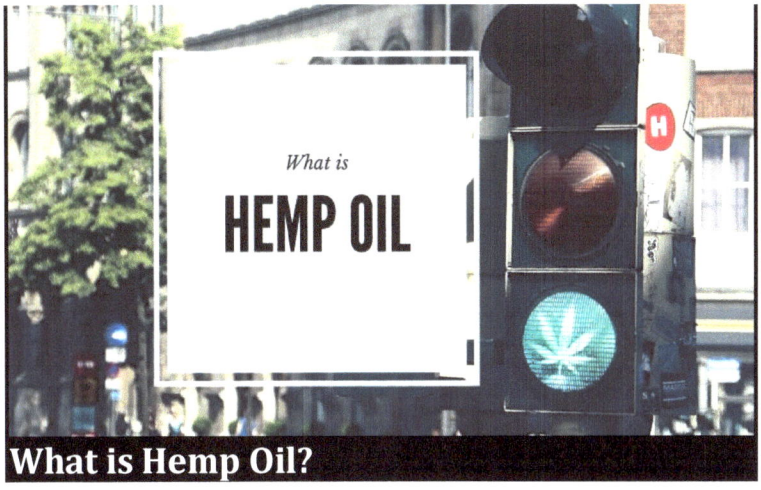

What is Hemp Oil?

First and foremost, where is hemp oil made from, where it can be found and how it is extracted.

This information is important, because these qualities distinguish it from the parent plant, marijuana.

One is legal, but the other is not, so such distinctions are useful.

To clarify hemp oil and marijuana come from the same plant.

However, hemp oil is extracted directly from the seeds.

It does not involve the leaves or stems of the plant, because these contain THC.

The difference still causes a lot of confusion for those in interested in the health benefits of hemp oil.

Not everybody is aware of the fact that you can't smoke or use hash oil (cannabis oil), but the non-psychotropic part of the plant is fine.

It has certainly impeded the widespread use of hemp oils in medical studies and trials.

Despite recommendations from doctors and leading medical researchers, the industry is still largely unwilling to work with hemp oil, due to its cultural and social associations with marijuana.

The best hemp oil comes from tall growing cannabis varieties, with low THC concentrations.

Depending on how it has been processed after it has left the plant, it can in many different forms. When cold pressed, but unfiltered, hemp oil is a dark green color and it is cloudy and dense.

It has a distinctly nutty flavor, with a hint of grass. On the other hand, filtered hemp oil has no color and a lot less flavor. It also lacks many of the nutrients contained in the original hemp seeds.

Ultimately, this means that the each variety can be used for different purposes.

If the hemp oil is needed for nutritional reasons (to improve general health or treat the symptoms of a chronic condition), unrefined oil is the best choice.

If it is being used for topical purposes (to treat a skin problem), refined products are more suitable.

The odor of both varieties is quite pungent, so it is best to keep hemp oil products in an air tight container, out of direct sunlight.

Hemp oil is filled with omega 6 and omega 3, both of which are essential for a healthy body and mind. It is also believed to have antibacterial, antioxidant, antiviral, antifungal, skin regenerative, cardio-protective, and anti-inflammatory properties.

If there's something missing, hemp oil is likely to provide it; that is how wide reaching its benefits are.

Luckily as the taboos around recreational marijuana are being toppled, so too are the obstacles preventing hemp oil from being fully investigated and researched.

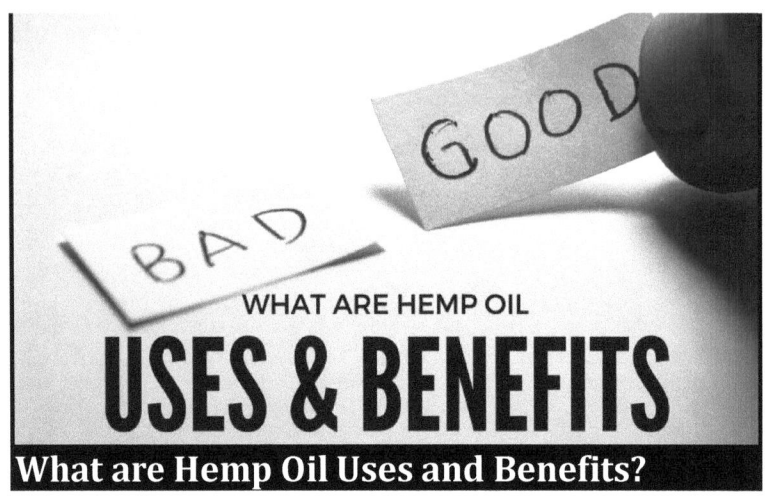

What are Hemp Oil Uses and Benefits?

The list of health benefits linked to hemp oil is so long that they can not all be featured here.

They include things such as a stronger immune system, healthier blood sugars, softer skin, a more robust nervous system, lower cholesterol, and a more stable hormonal balance, to name a few.

The nutritional use of hemp oil is widely believed to improve cancer symptoms, alleviate anxiety and solve both minor and major dietary deficiencies.

It is important to note that, while these health benefits are very compelling and of great interest to medical researchers, there is still a distinct lack of formal, repeatable medical studies on hemp oil.

As discussed, this is largely because of its association with the marijuana plant.

The illegality of marijuana has prevented decades of perfectly legal and legitimate studies from taking place, simply because the taboo is strong enough to deter funding and sponsorship.

The good news is that things are changing. Over the last twenty years, the number of medical studies on hemp oil have soared and scientists are starting to build up an accurate picture of the benefits.

One of the most fascinating claims is that hemp oil may be effective at preventing even serious degenerative diseases such as cancer.

There is evidence to suggest that the nutritional balance of omega 3 fats and prostaglandins (a hormone nurturing substance) can keep cancer at bay, if used as a dietary supplement.

According to the British Journal of Cancer, hemp seeds have the potential to stop and, rather remarkably, reverse the symptoms of glioblastoma multiforme (a fatal form of brain cancer).

This claim is supported by the Journal of Breast Cancer Research and Treatment, which has also found evidence to suggest that hemp seeds can improve the symptoms of advanced stage breast cancer.

These are, by no means, the only medical studies to make such claims, so it seems clear to see that hemp oil and hemp seeds are extremely valuable.

Hemp oil has also been linked to improvements in anxiety disorders, which may sound strange to anybody with a knowledge of marijuana.

However, while the THC in marijuana does tend to cause paranoia and anxiety, in large enough does, the CBD in hemp oil actually counteracts these responses.

As it has intensely anxiolytic properties, hemp oil actively keeps stress and anxiety at bay.

This has made it a focus of research for scientists studying mood disorders and trying to find treatments for sufferers of chronic anxiety.

The benefits for hair and skin are impressive. Fatty acids are extremely good for the skin and hemp oil is filled with them.

They nourish and moisturize, without being abrasive or drying out the pores. Conditions like eczema, psoriasis, chronic acne, and persistent dry skin have all been treated with hemp oil.

Lastly, there are the benefits for hair.

Washing with hemp oil enhances blood circulation to the scalp, thickens follicles, and treats dandruff.

There is evidence to suggest that the rate of hair loss can be slowed with the use of hemp oils.

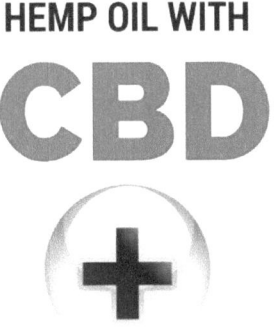

HEMP OIL WITH CBD

Hemp Oil with CBD

There is a huge amount of confusion around the distinction between hemp oil and CBD oil. The misconceptions surrounding both are abundant.

This is, perhaps, unsurprising because the difference (though important) is a fairly subtle one. As the taboo around all products associated with the marijuana plant remains strong, people still feel like they are not allowed to ask questions.

This makes them vulnerable to unscrupulous suppliers and dealers who are not too concerned about whether customers get exactly the right product.

The distinction is important, however, so keep it in mind when shopping for hemp oil products in the future. While hemp oil is derived from crushed hemp seeds, CBD oil is primarily extracted from the hemp flowers, leaves, and stalks.

As far as composition, it contains a much higher amount of the chemical compound, CBD (cannabidiol), than hemp oil does. Crucially, neither hemp oil nor CBD oil contains enough THC to get a person high.

Essentially, CBD oil is kind of like regular hemp oil, but with all of the associated benefits tripled. Hemp is its gentler, softer relative.

This is why it is easy to find hemp oil in high street stores. It is contained in everything from hand lotions to shampoo, face creams, cosmetics and anti-aging products. As CBD oil is much stronger, it is much more likely to be used in medical trials and studies.

Where hemp is ubiquitous these days, CBD is still treated with a lot of suspicion. In most countries, including the US, it is legal but there are some grey areas around its distribution and sales.

Nevertheless, it is legal to use CBD oils, as long as they do not contain anything but trace amounts of THC.

They cannot get a person high, but they may be used to treat all of the conditions already discussed.

They may also be used to alleviate the symptoms of mood disorders and chronic anxiety.

The popularity of CBD oils has soared in recent years, despite the persistent confusion around their use, and the market for CBD vape oils and related products continues to grow at a rapid rate.

It is very important, for anybody interested in buying hemp or CBD oils, that the distinction between the two is recognized and understood.

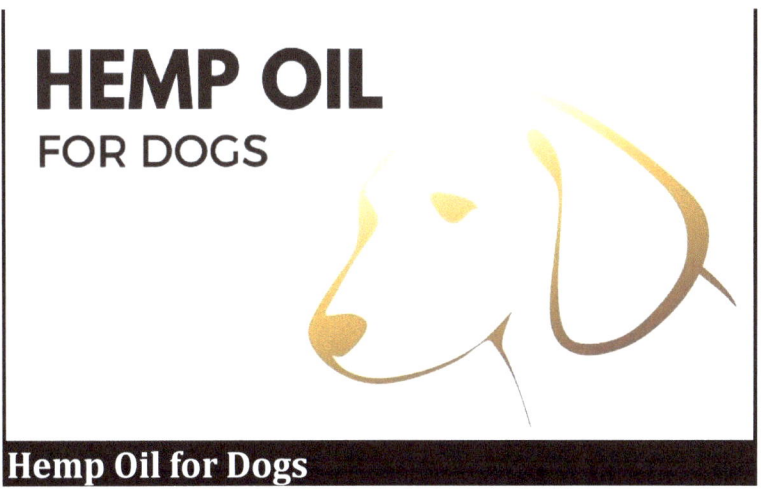

Hemp Oil for Dogs

It may come as a surprise to find that the benefits of hemp oil are not limited to humans. In fact, there is compelling evidence to suggest that it is hugely advantageous for canines too.

Many of the nutritional and health benefits of hemp oil for humans also apply to dogs. For instance, pets who suffer with cancer, diabetes, or skin allergies (like humans) don't produce enough GLA (an essential fatty acid) and hemp oil supplements are an easy way to solve this problem.

They reduce inflammation and give the immune system a substantial boost.

Once again, hemp oil has no THC and does not produce any psychotropic properties.

If it is bought as a natural product, with no other added chemicals, it poses no harm for dogs whatsoever.

However, just one teaspoon per day is more than enough, even for large pets.

Supplementation with hemp seed oil supports good heart health, improves the condition of the skin and fur, reduces the rate of shedding, encourages healthy organ function, and has a positive impact on brain health and development.

There are a couple of things to remember before adding hemp oil to a canine diet. The first is that it should never be cooked.

It is a polyunsaturated fat, so it cannot be heated or it will turn rancid.

This is dangerous for the health of both pets and humans, so hemp oil should always be added after cooking food. It is also worth remembering that diets already high in protein (particularly chicken and turkey) may lead to nutritional imbalances if hemp oil is added as well.

This is because both poultry and hemp oil are very high in linoleic acid and healthy fats.

It may be a better idea for these diets to be supplemented with flaxseed oil instead of hemp oil, so that the volumes of both remain stable.

Otherwise, there are no dangers or risks associated with the supplementation of canine diets with hemp oil.

The benefits are numerous and medical researchers are continuing to build up a clear picture of this wonder substance.

In the years to come, there will be more studies and, hopefully, the reputation of hemp oil will be celebrated and restored.

For those who are interested in trying hemp oil, either for its nutritional benefits or its ability to relax and calm an anxious mind, it is important to remember that the substance comes in a wide variety of forms.

It can be bought and used as a tincture. It can also be ingested as capsules. It may even be bought as a protein powder. Or, alternatively, 'hemp oil' can be picked up as seeds, before it is actually turned into oil.

With so many choices on offer, people can pick the type of application that best suits their lifestyle.

For instance, if the main priority is healthier skin, the best option is to pick up a topical cream with hemp oil in the formula.

If anxiety is the biggest concern, oral capsules are likely to be the most effective choice, because they are fast acting and easy to take. It is a good idea to exercise caution when shopping, because it can be tricky to pick the right product.

All hemp oil products should be bought from a reputable dealer, with a license to trade cannabidiol compounds.

It is still very much illegal to smoke or consume THC, so make sure that purchases contain hemp oil and not cannabis oil.

There is no THC in hemp oil, which means that it does not have any psychotropic properties.

It will not get a person high, but it may induce feelings of relaxation and calm.

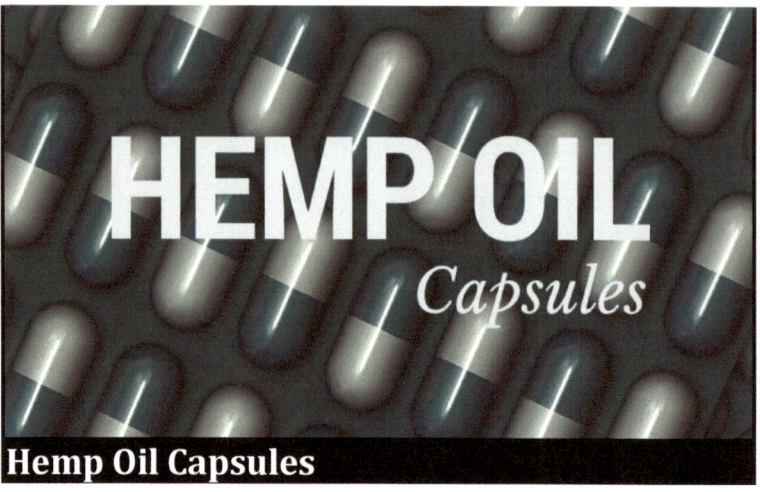

Hemp Oil Capsules

The easiest way to boost general health and take advantage of the nutritional benefits of hemp oil is by taking dietary hemp oil capsules.

There are endless advantages to consuming hemp oil in this way.

It is not only fast and efficient, it is discreet too.

For those who are not entirely comfortable with ingesting CBD compounds publically, capsules provide greater control and privacy.

They can, quite literally, be popped in the mouth within seconds, just like any other supplement.

While raw hemp oil continues to be a popular choice, there are lots of people who simply don't like the taste.

Capsules are the ideal solution, because they produce no flavor at all if they are swallowed whole, as recommended.

They also make it easier for users to monitor the amount of CBD that is being consumed.

Every capsule contains exactly the same amount of high grade cannabidiol, so it's pretty difficult to accidentally exceed the advised dosage.

The type of hemp oil found in dietary capsules is no different to that which is sold as pure or raw oil.

The distinction is in how it is packaged; hemp oil capsules are enclosed inside soft glycerine shells that break down in the stomach after they have been swallowed.

They are particularly well suited to users who are interested in enhancing their overall health.

Taking one to two capsules per day will improve the condition of skin and hair, regulate hormone levels, lower cholesterol, and aid cardiovascular circulation and organ health.

They are also a good choice for people who are new to hemp oil and aren't yet sure what type of products they should buy.

Taking the exact same amount, every time, is beneficial, because it provides a much more stable and predictable outcome.

With hemp oil capsules, users know exactly what they're getting each time that they take a dose.

They come in a range of different sizes and strengths, so it's important to shop carefully.

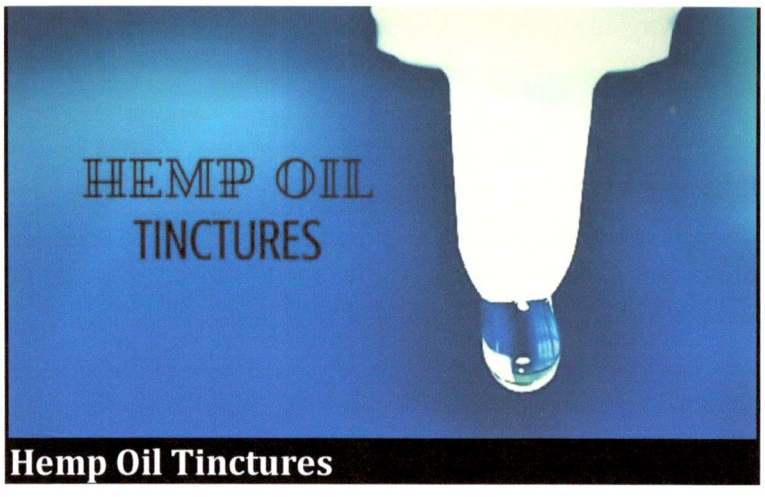

Hemp Oil Tinctures

However, capsules aren't the only way to benefit from the remarkable properties of hemp oil.

It can also be bought in the form of tinctures. In fact, this is one of the most popular ways to use hemp oil, because it is just as easy as swallowing a capsule, but it provides a stronger, faster acting dose.

With a tincture, the oil is applied directly to the tongue or throat, from a dropper style bottle.

Like capsules, tinctures are as discreet as users want to make them, because the small containers fit neatly into a pocket or handbag.

Hemp oil tinctures are recommended for users who are already comfortable and familiar with these products.

They may not be the best choice for new users, because the average dose is significantly stronger in a tincture than it is in a capsule.

They make an effective treatment for anxiety, as the hemp oil drops are activated almost immediately.

Some vendors sell their tinctures in spray bottles, instead of containers with dropper tops, but the application is the same in either case.

Spray bottle tinctures are easy to use and very convenient.

They also make monitoring dosage simple, because every spray of the bottle contains a specific amount of oil (and CBD).

Plus, tinctures can be flavored, which makes them more appealing than raw oils.

For those who struggle to swallow pills or tablets, this option provides a no fuss solution.

Do be aware that many of these products are made with alcohol.

There are alcohol free versions available, but they may have to be bought from a supplier who specializes in all natural hemp oil products.

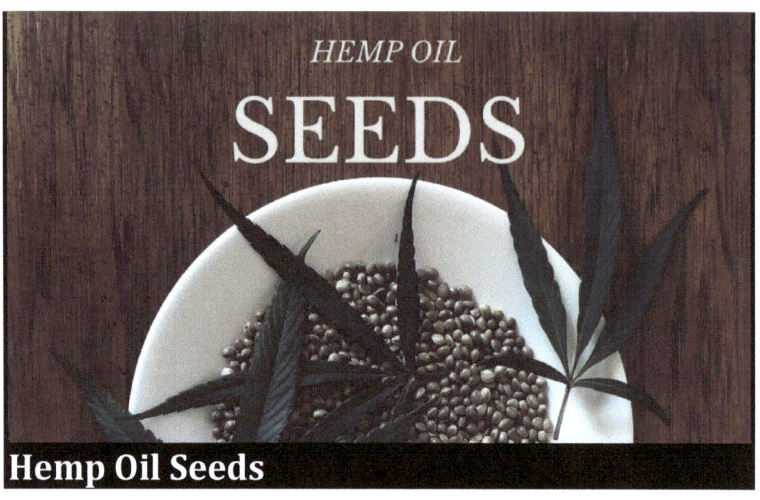

Hemp Oil Seeds

It is also possible to buy and consume organic hemp oil seeds, but this is a less common option.

It is generally only recommended for those who want to benefit from the nutritional value of hemp oil, without actually consuming pure oil.

Hemp Oil seeds should not be used for cooking, however, as the heat makes the oil rancid.

They can be eaten, but they must be eaten raw, on the top of things like cereals, granola, and salads. Or, they can, of course, just be eaten on their own as a healthy snack.

They are a fantastic way to boost nutrition, because they contain all of the essential amino acids.

Plus, 65% of the protein found in hemp oil seeds is in a substance called globulin edistin.

It is a basic protein, but it gives the body everything that it needs to produce the immunoglobulins necessary for fighting off sickness and infections.

As the human body can't naturally create its own globulin edistin, the only way to get enough is to eat foods that contain it in high volumes, like hemp seeds.

In China, they have been eaten for thousands of years as a traditional food.

This is actually where most of the hemp seed products sold in health food stores originally come from. Crucially, consuming hemp seeds does not get a person high, nor will it cause them to fail a drugs test.

There is only a negligible amount of THC in these seeds; no more than is contained in poppy seeds, for example.

As hemp seeds have an earthy, nutty flavor, they are a great substitute for people who are allergic to nuts.

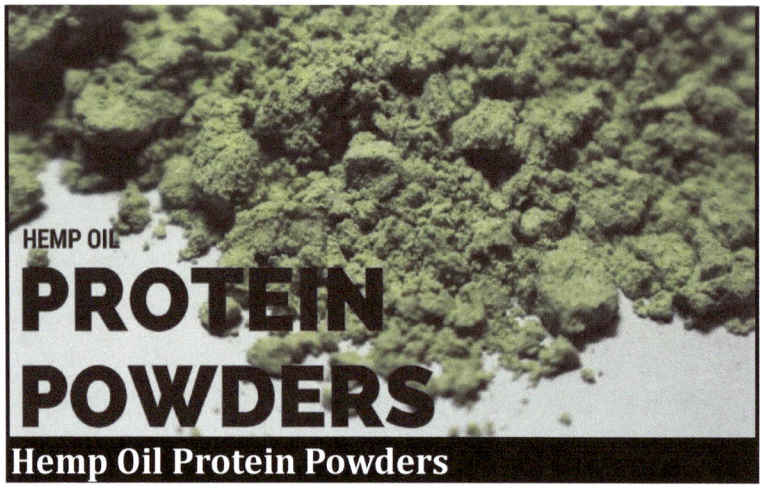

Hemp Oil Protein Powders

While tinctures, raw oils, and capsules are very common choices, most users aren't aware that it is also possible to buy hemp oil protein powders.

These formulas are a nutritional supplement; they can be consumed in things like smoothies and baked goods.

At around 15g of protein per serving (on average), hemp based powders are not only powerfully nourishing, they are completely natural too.

This makes them a suitable choice for vegetarians, particularly those who struggle to find suitable supplements and dietary powders.

Hemp Oil protein powders of all kinds are a popular choice with athletes and bodybuilders, because they encourage the accelerated repair of lean body mass.

Hemp contains an abundance of branched amino acids and these play an important part in the growth and regeneration of muscle.

Plus, hemp is also rich in the sulfur containing amino acids, cysteine and methionine; they are both essential for the healthy production of enzymes.

Hemp based protein powders are easy to consume and digest, but they are not the best option for those in need of a fast acting response.

They take a little longer to get to work than capsules or tinctures, but when they do, the impact is robust and sustained.

With its pleasantly nutty flavor and aroma, this eco-friendly superfood is another great way to take advantage of the health and nutritional benefits of hemp oil.

For a truly natural product, make sure that the protein powder does not contain any gluten or additional sugars.

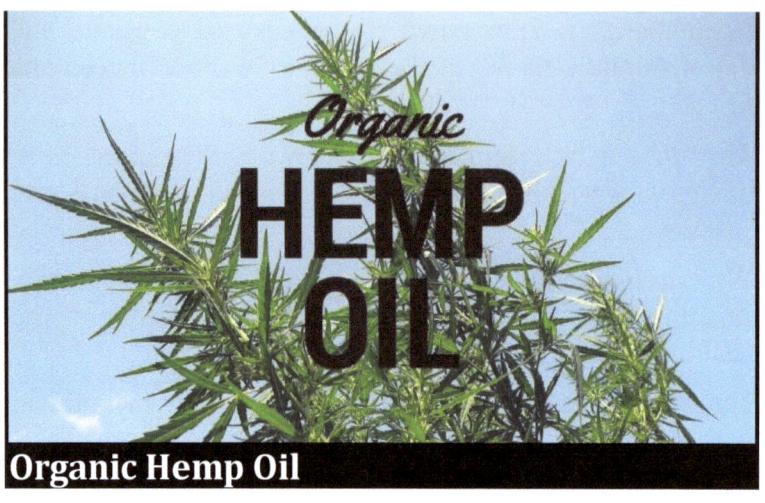

Organic Hemp Oil

Finally, the health benefits of hemp may also be enjoyed in the form of organic hemp culinary oils. It is important to note that these products can only be used for low heat cooking or consumed raw; cooking at a high heat will cause the oil to turn rancid and make it unsuitable for eating.

However, organic hemp oil is ideal for drizzling over salads, stir fries, potatoes, pasta dishes, vegetables, and more. It is also particularly tasty when used as a raw dip for crusty bread.

The flavor is earthy and nutty, but very smooth. It lends itself well to smoothies, fruit juices, shakes, and yoghurts.

All organic hemp oil products should be cold pressed and unrefined, because too much processing destroys the nutritional value of the seeds and they end up having a much milder effect on the body.

It needs to be kept refrigerated and consumed within four months, after opening.

Therefore, anybody looking to buy a hemp oil product that will last is advised to opt for capsules or tinctures instead.

They have a longer shelf life and may be used as a dietary supplement, over a prolonged period.

Organic hemp oils are suitable for vegetarian diets and those with sensitive digestive systems, because they are kind to the stomach and organs.

They are rich in protein, omega fatty acids, and fiber, as well as all twenty essential amino acids.

This form of hemp oil is just another example of how diverse the substance can be. It doesn't have to be eaten raw; it can be added to a whole variety of different ingredients and compounds to create something that is as tasty as it is nutritious.

To reiterate, CBD hemp oil is a dietary supplement made from industrial hemp. It is available in all US states. No permit or prescription is needed to purchase CBD hemp oil products.

However, it's important to be an informed consumer, because there are lots of different varieties on offer.

CBD hemp oil should only be bought from a reputable vendor, with all of the licenses and qualifications needed to sell these compounds legally and commercially.

It should be clear by now that the benefits of hemp oil are endless and continue to grow as medical researchers and scientists get to know them better.

Over the coming decade, it is inevitable that we will see more research into the impact of CBD and hemp oils and this may lead to a change in attitudes across society.

At the moment, the association that hemp oil has with cannabis (or marijuana) can hamper attempts to study it.

For now, there is much evidence to suggest that hemp oil is a super substance; a nutritional compound that all but eclipses every other dietary supplement on the market when it comes to health boosting properties.

It can be consumed and applied in a huge variety of ways – everything from salad dressings to topical ointments, shampoos, and tinctures – and this makes it suitable for just about anybody.

Those who are completely new to CBD and hemp oils might want to try one of the milder forms first and move on to things like tinctures later.

For a first experience, organic oils and pure hemp seeds are a good choice, because they can be eaten in small amounts and added to regular meals.

Plus, the taste is pleasant and may actually enhance the flavor of vegetables, pasta dishes, rice, and more.

To get the most out of any hemp oil product, it needs to be stored carefully, according to the guidance provided by the manufacturer.

Source - http://cannabiscbdoil.org

www.ingramcontent.com/pod-product-compliance
Lightning Source LLC
Chambersburg PA
CBHW050927290526
45792CB00002B/919